Paleo Diet For Beginners: 7-Day Paleo Meal Plan with Healthy & Delicious Recipes for the Ultimate Primal Diet

Nina Bookes

Wait! Before you read on I would love to share a couple of free gifts with you as a thank you for purchasing this book.

These bonus gifts contain additional healthy, mouth-watering Paleo recipes along with a great work out guide to help you on your journey and teach you how to maintain your weight once you lose it. Grab your copies today absolutely FREE! See the last chapter for details.

accepted and approved equally by a Committee of the American Bar Association and a Committee of Publishers and Associations.

Table of Contents

Paleo Diet For Beginners

Introduction

I want to thank you and congratulate you for downloading the book, "Paleo Diet for Beginners: 7-Day Paleo Meal Plan with Healthy & Delicious Recipes".

Are you constantly struggling to make a positive and healthier change in your eating habits? If your answer is yes then this book is just what you need, as it contains proven steps and strategies on how to create a 7-day meal plan based on the principles of the Paleo Diet. It is a lifestyle change, which mainly focuses on using clean, organic ingredients to create delicious meals that nourish the body, mind and spirit.

The term "paleo," which refers to caveman-like traits, was coined by Dr. Loren Cordain, an exercise physiologist who first published a book on this revolutionary diet program in 2002. In his extensive research, Dr. Cordain discovered how prehistoric man survived on a diet that's free of grains, dairy and other agriculturally-processed food. This discovery led him to create a diet, which is rich of organic ingredients that contain natural vitamins and minerals.

The paleo diet is the perfect program for you if you want to change your life for the better by just using basic nutrition know-how. Its principles promote the consumption of organic food items such as fruits, vegetables, eggs, healthy oils, protein, nuts and seeds that are all genetically familiar to the human body. Adding these foods to your daily meals will make it easier for you to lose weight, have a stronger immune system and achieve a better quality of life.

As you go through the chapters of this book, you will be presented with basic yet essential information about the Paleo Diet, including its beginnings, health benefits, a complete Paleo-friendly food guide, and a list of food substitutions that will help you make paleo-friendly replacements to processed, unhealthy ingredients.

Moreover, the 7-day meal plan in this book contains over 40 recipes ranging from breakfast, lunch, dinner, snack and dessert.

These dishes are made from fresh and clean ingredients, such as organic vegetables, fruits, meats, eggs, herbs, spices, grain-free flours and healthy oils that are readily available in local markets and groceries. These recipes will prove to you how easy and enjoyable cooking can be while following a cleaner paleo lifestyle.

Paleo Diet: A Primitive Approach to Modern-day Nutrition

"One cannot think well, love well and sleep well if he has not dined well."

Virginia Woolf

Taking inspiration from the ancient eating habits and cooking methods of pre-agricultural man, the Paleo Diet encourages people to appreciate the simplicity of consuming organic food, which has either spurted from the earth or sourced from animals such as cows, chicken or fish. Eating paleo-friendly foods that the human body is accustomed to can help you achieve a slimmer and disease-free body and a better quality of life.

Before we discuss the details behind this caveman-like approach towards nutrition, let us understand how this diet program started and why it has influenced people to be more aware of their eating habits.

Dr. Lauren Cordain and the Paleo Movement

In 1987, Dr. Loren Cordain, an exercise physiologist and researcher of the Colorado State University stumbled upon a published manuscript entitled "Paleolithic Nutrition: a Consideration of its Nature and Current Implications" written by Dr. Boyd Eaton. This science paper stirred Cordain's interest in prehistoric nutrition and its effects on the human body.

In his paleo-themed manuscript, Dr. Cordain found out that prehistoric man survived its hunting and gathering activities without the need to eat grains. They mainly survived on animal meat, water, plants and seeds. This discovery triggered Cordain to read more than 25,000 scientific manuscripts on the Paleo diet over the next eight years.

Based on Dr. Cordain's extensive research, he concluded that Paleolithic man survived the world without consuming grains, dairy and other agriculturally processed foods.

Moreover, past scientific studies show how modern-day foods contributed to the declining health of non-westernized groups, such as Indians, Eskimos and African tribes, once they were exposed to these products.

All these scientific facts supported Dr. Cordain's development of the paleo diet program, which caused him to publish "The Paleo Diet" in 2002. In this book, Cordain discusses how the paleo diet is a low-glycemic and high-protein program, which promotes weight loss, disease cure & prevention and better blood chemistry.

Over the years, scientists have tested Dr. Cordain's paleo principles and came up with favorable results. Dr. Kerin O-Dea of the University of Melbourne created a study wherein tribal people were exposed to processed foods over a certain period, resulting to them becoming obese, sedentary and diabetic. When the same people were asked to revert back to their paleo lifestyle, their cholesterol, insulin and triglyceride numbers went down.

In another experiment, Dr. Staffan Lindeberg

of Lund University, Sweden made a group of diabetics undergo the paleo diet for 3 months and a diabetic diet for the next 3 months. Results showed that when patients followed a paleo meal plan, they had better health and lower numbers in terms of waist size, weight, blood sugar, cholesterol and hemoglobin.

The results of these experiments and advanced studies about human diets prove that the principles Dr. Cordain created for the paleo are definitely true and life-changing, as it may help cure both simple and complex diseases that threaten man's longevity.

Principles of the Paleo Diet

The paleo diet encourages people to stick to a diet, which is free of sugars, salty foods, GMOs and other processed items. Here are the basic principles to follow if you want to embrace this healthy and life-changing diet program:

1. Eat more of low-carbohydrate and low-glycemic foods

Carbohydrates from foods such as breads, sugars and potatoes are high in glycemic index, causing blood sugar levels to reach dangerous, disease-causing levels. Lessening your carb intake and eating more plant-based foods will help regulate your insulin levels and hormones, which in turn prevents weight gain, diabetes and other serious medical conditions.

2. Increase intake of fiber

Dietary fiber from green leafy vegetables and other non-starchy plants can easily replace the fiber found in unhealthy grains. In fact, fruits and vegetables contain 8-10 times more fiber than wheat bread or brown rice. Based on these findings, it is safe to conclude that consuming paleo foods will not only make you feel full, but can also help your body achieve healthy digestion.

3. Increase intake of protein

Meats, poultry and fish should make up at least 20-30% of the calories in an average man's daily diet. Protein is what made our prehistoric ancestors thrive in a grain-free diet. High consumption of protein allows the stomach to feel full for longer periods while also building muscle tissues during physically strenuous activities.

4. Increase consumption of good fats

Consuming good fats such as olive oil, avocados and coconuts are not harmful to the body. These monounsaturated fats promote weight loss, bone health, mental balance, heart health and longevity. Moreover, the dietary fat from these healthy oils is easily converted to energy, which is essential in performing weight loss activities, such as weight training and aerobics.

5. Lower the salt and increase potassium

Both potassium and salt have serious but different impact on your kidneys, heart and other organs. Paleo foods are normally low in sodium and high in potassium, thus, they can prevent the occurrence of heart ailments,

urinary tract infections and other degenerative diseases.

6. Balanced high-acid foods with high-alkaline vegetables and fruits

Plant-based items, such as fruits and vegetables have high alkaline content, which greatly balances the acidity of foods, such as fatty fish. A healthy balance of acid and.

Health Benefits of a Paleo Lifestyle

Transitioning to a healthier paleo lifestyle is worth every minute of your time and effort because of its positively life-changing effects on your health. Here are the health benefits that paleo advocates have experienced as a result of making better food choices and changing unhealthy eating habits:

- Long-term weight management

- Lean muscle formation

- Improved fat cell burning ability

- Improved mental health

- Clearer skin and shinier hair

- Stronger immune system

- Lower risk of having serious diseases such as diabetes, heart ailments and cancer

Lower blood sugar and cholesterol levels

Regulated blood pressure levels

Healthy cell production and organ maintenance

Improved digestion

Reduce or eliminate stomach conditions

Lesser allergies

Better sleep patterns

Higher energy levels needed for daily activities

Now that we know the positive effects of eating paleo-friendly foods, it is time to identify the foods that support this healthier lifestyle and those that you should avoid completely.

Complete Paleo Diet Food Guide for Beginners

If you want to begin a new paleo lifestyle, it is essential to have basic know-how about the diet such as its guiding principles, health benefits and the right type of ingredients to cook with. It is vital to use organic and nutritious ingredients when cooking paleo, so that you can train your mind to create healthier dishes that your body can positively respond to.

The following food list will serve as your guide when shopping for paleo-friendly food items:

What to Eat on Paleo

A paleo diet promotes organic, free-range food items that are rich in vitamins, minerals and flavor.

Meats – beef, chicken, turkey, goose, lamb, duck, ostrich, sheep, deer, bison, reindeer, pheasant, quail, elk, kangaroo.

Animal organs – liver, kidney, tongue, marrow, sweetbreads.

Fish and Seafood – lobster, scallops, shrimp, clams, mussels, oysters, salmon, bass, tilapia, sardines, halibut, tuna, mackerel, shark, swordfish, red snapper, flatfish, trout, sole, anchovy, haddock, herring, walleye.

Leafy Vegetables – kale, collard greens, Swiss chard, spinach, lettuce, bok choy, arugula, cabbage, watercress, chicory, turnip greens, mustard greens, beet greens.

Other Vegetables – broccoli, tomatoes, zucchini, bell peppers, celery, turnips, carrots, cucumber, leeks, scallions, cauliflower, okra, avocado, artichokes, Brussels sprouts, eggplants, radish, beets, sweet potatoes, pumpkin, squash.
Note: Eat starchy vegetables such as squash, sweet potatoes and pumpkin in moderation .

Eggs – chicken eggs, duck eggs, goose eggs, quail eggs, ostrich eggs.

Fruits – lemon, pineapple, lime, mango, apple, orange, banana, watermelon, melon, strawberry, blueberry, raspberry, blackberry, lychee, kiwi, cherry, pear, grapefruit, peach,

apricot, plum, nectarine, tangerine, grapes, papaya, passion fruit, dates, olives
Note: Consume high-sugar fruits such as berries in moderation.

Mushrooms – button, cremini, shiitake, porcini, oyster, portobello, morel, chanterelle.

Oils – olive oil, coconut oil, avocado oil, sesame oil, walnut oil, macadamia oil, grass-fed butter, ghee, nut butters, lard.

Nuts & Seeds – almond, pecan, walnut, macadamia, pistachio, Brazil nuts, hazelnut, chestnut, cashew, chia seeds, flaxseed meal, pumpkin seeds, sunflower seeds.

Herbs – parsley, coriander, thyme, sage, rosemary, mint, oregano, marjoram, dill, basil, bay leaves.

Spices – sea salt, peppercorns, garlic, ginger, chili peppers, paprika, cumin, nutmeg, cinnamon, cayenne, chili flakes, turmeric, vanilla, cloves.

Drinks – water, natural and unsweetened fruit juice, black coffee, herbal tea, coconut water, natural fruit and vegetable smoothies, dairy-free milk blends.

Condiments – vinegar, mustard, organic mayonnaise, paleo ketchup, coconut aminos.

Others – coconut milk, almond milk, coconut flesh, almond flour, coconut flour, tapioca flour, arrowroot flour, coconut sugar, organic honey, maple syrup, stevia, vanilla extract, almond extract, cocoa powder, baking powder, baking soda.

What Not to Eat on Paleo

Foods that do not support the paleo principles include high-carb vegetables, grains, GMOs, manufactured meals, fast food items, artificial sugars and processed meats.

Starchy Vegetables – potatoes, plantains, yucca, corn.

Legumes – soy, soy beans, soy sauce, tofu, peas, chickpeas, peanuts, beans.

Processed Meat – hotdogs, salami, ham, pepperoni, canned meats.

Dairy – all types of cheese, milk, margarine, creamer, yoghurt, ice cream, dairy spreads.

Drinks – soft drinks, fruit juices, coffee

blends, sweetened teas, energy drinks, vodka, tequila, beer, rum, whiskey.

Sweets – candies, chocolate bars, jams, sugary cereals, high-sugar energy bars, cookies, artificial sweeteners, corn syrup, table sugar.

Grains – rice, wheat, quinoa, all-purpose flour, bread, sandwiches, crackers, muffins, pancake mix, baking mix, instant oatmeal, pasta, cupcakes, pastries, croutons.

Instant Foods & Snacks – hash browns, chips, frozen meals, packaged nuts, pretzels, popcorn, fries, burgers, fast-food items.

Others – table salt, canola oil, vegetable oil, sunflower oil.

This food list will help you get rid of unhealthy and processed foods from the kitchen and empower you to make smarter choices when buying ingredients from the grocery or market.

Initially, you may find it difficult to alter certain recipes into becoming paleo friendly, but this food list shows that going paleo gives you healthier options for ingredients that are good for the body. In case you may have a favorite recipe, there are healthy paleo substitutes that will still allow you to enjoy it.

Top 15 Paleo-Friendly Food Substitutions

The paleo diet is a flexible diet program because it allows healthier ingredient replacements without losing the flavor and texture of certain dishes. Here are 15 paleo substitutes that you can use to create delectable yet healthy meals in the kitchen:

1. *Cauliflower*

Instead of rice, potatoes

How to use: Grind cauliflower into smaller grains in a food processor then fry in butter. Boil or stir-fry cauliflower florets for stews, omelets and salads.

2. *Coconut aminos*

Instead of soy sauce, Worcestershire sauce, oyster sauce

How to use: Place a few drops of this paleo-friendly and gluten-free seasoning when doing vegetable stir-fries, marinades or crock pot stews.

3. Dark Chocolate

Instead of milk chocolate

How to use: Melt dark chocolate squares or chips in a double boiler then use when baking brownies, cakes and puddings. Chop coarsely then fold into cookie or muffin batter.

4. Coconut sugar, honey or maple syrup

Instead of regular sugar, artificial sweeteners

How to use: Blend into dessert, snack and drink recipes in place of regular sugar or artificial alternatives.

5. Ground nuts and seeds

Instead of bread crumbs, breading mixes

How to use: Place nuts or seeds in a food processor then process for 30-60 seconds until the texture is similar to regular bread crumbs. You can dredge chicken, fish or other protein into this breading mixture then fry it.

6. *Nutritional yeast*

Instead of cheese, thickening agents

How to use: Place a thin layer of nutritional yeast on top of dishes that conventionally require melted cheese. Place a few teaspoons while boiling sauces for a thicker consistency.

7. *Almond milk or coconut milk*

Instead of pasteurized cow's milk

How to use: Use either almond or coconut milk when creating sauces, chowders or curry dishes. Blend milk into wet ingredients for cakes, cookies, muffins or puddings. Pour milk into breakfast oats or cereals

8. *Almond flour or coconut flour*

Instead of all-purpose flour, cake flour

How to use: Incorporate these Paleo flours into recipes for cookies, pies, cupcakes or muffins. Use flour as breading for fish, chicken and other meats.

9. *Sea salt*

Instead of iodized salt

How to use: Sprinkle sea salt in salad dressings, soups, main dishes, snacks and breakfast dishes.

10. *Organic vegetables*

Instead of: chemically-grown vegetables

How to use: Chop, mash, boil, stir-fry, roast or eat raw – the culinary possibilities with vegetables are endless .

11. *Zucchini or raw vegetable noodles*

Instead of pasta

How to use: Cut vegetables such as zucchini, beets or sweet potatoes through a spiralizer until long, noodle-like strands are produced. Stir-fry, boil or toss these noodles with your favorite pasta sauce.

12. *Sweet potatoes*

Instead of potatoes

How to use: To make chips, slice sweet potatoes into thin layers then bake. Boil then mash sweet potatoes for pies, puddings, soups and stews.

13. Homemade Paleo breads

Instead of regular bread

How to use: Make your own paleo breads, biscuits, crackers and muffins using almond flour or coconut flour then serve along soups, salads or breakfast dishes.

14. Homemade vegetable chips/fries

Instead of potato chips, fries

How to use: Chop leafy greens such as kale or collard greens then bake until crisp. Slice carrots or turnips into long sticks then bake.

15. Coconut oil or olive oil

Instead of vegetable oil, canola oil, margarine

How to use: Pour oil in pan to fry   meats, eggs and vegetables. Mix oils with vinegar's to create salad dressings. Blend oil with chocolate or coconut milk for paleo-friendly desserts.

Now that you have a complete list of ingredients, as well as popular paleo-friendly replacements, you can start planning your meals around the principles of the paleo diet with minimal effort.

Day 1 - Dairy-Free Breakfast Waffles

Creating a meal plan with the paleo principles in mind can be hassle-free once you have a collection of nutrient-dense recipes that range from breakfast, lunch, dinner, snack and dessert. However, keep in mind that a healthy ratio of protein, fats and carbohydrates is essential in reaping the benefits of a paleo lifestyle.

Here is a 7-day paleo meal plan for you to start with:

Breakfast

Dairy-Free Breakfast Waffles

Ingredients:

1 cup almond flour

2 tablespoons coconut flour

2 teaspoons coconut sugar

2 large eggs

2 teaspoons baking powder

½ teaspoon apple cider vinegar

1 tablespoon olive oil

7 tablespoons almond milk

Directions:

Preheat the waffle maker and place a little cooking spray on the waffle tins.

Mix almond flour, coconut flour, coconut sugar and baking powder in a bowl. Set aside.

In a separate bowl, whisk the eggs together with the olive oil, almond milk and apple cider vinegar. Pour the mixture into the bowl of dry ingredients and mix well.

Pour the waffle batter into the waffle maker and close it. Let the waffles cook for 4 minutes or until golden brown. Transfer the waffles to a plate and serve immediately.

This recipe makes 4 servings.

Note: In case you do not have a waffle maker, just pour the batter into a greased frying pan. Fry each batter until brown on both sides to create pancakes out of the same recipe.

Nutrition: 250 calories; 6g carbohydrates; 25g fats; 20g protein

Tangy Asparagus Chicken Skillet with Roasted Carrots

Lunch

Ingredients:

350g chicken breast, skin removed and cubed

1 large carrot, peeled and julienned

1 cup chopped asparagus

1 teaspoon white vinegar

3 teaspoons olive oil

1 teaspoon dried rosemary

½ teaspoon garlic powder

½ teaspoon lemon juice

½ teaspoon lemon zest

1 tablespoon almond flour

½ cup homemade chicken stock

1 teaspoon minced garlic

Pinch of salt and ground black pepper

Directions:

Place the chicken cubes in a bowl then add the flour, salt, pepper, lemon zest and garlic powder. Mix the ingredients until the chicken pieces are evenly coated.

Heat 2 teaspoons of olive oil in a skillet over medium-high flame. Cook the chicken in the skillet for 3 minutes or until the pieces turn light brown. Remove the chicken from the pan and set aside.

Add the garlic and asparagus into the skillet and cook for 3 minutes. Pour in the stock and vinegar then stir. Place the chicken back into the skillet, lower the heat to medium then cover the pan. Simmer the dish for 15 minutes.

While the dish is simmering, place the remaining olive oil, rosemary and carrots in a bowl then toss them together. Place the carrots in a parchment-lined pan and bake it in the oven under 350°F for 15 minutes. Once the carrots are tender, remove them from the oven and let them cool for 10 minutes.

Once the chicken is cooked, squeeze the lemon juice into the pan and stir. Turn off the flame and transfer the dish to a serving plate. Arrange the roasted carrots on the side and serve immediately.

This recipe makes 2 servings.

Nutrition: 260 calories; 20g carbohydrates; 6g fats; 40g protein

Hi-Fiber Zuccarot Muffins

Snack

Ingredients:

½ cup shredded zucchini

½ cup shredded carrots

6 tablespoons coconut flour

1 tablespoon flaxseed meal

½ cup coconut sugar

3 eggs

½ teaspoon apple cider vinegar

2 tablespoons coconut oil

¼ cup coconut milk

1 teaspoon cinnamon powder

1 ½ teaspoon baking powder

¼ teaspoon baking soda

1 teaspoon vanilla extract

Directions:

Preheat the oven to 350°F and place liners inside 12 muffin tins.

Combine coconut flour, coconut sugar, baking soda, baking powder, flaxseed meal and cinnamon powder in a bowl. Mix well.

In a separate bowl, blend together zucchini, carrots, vanilla extract, apple cider vinegar, eggs, coconut oil and coconut milk. Pour the wet ingredients into the bowl of dry ingredients and mix well.

Fill each muffin tin with the batter, making sure to leave 1/3 space on top. Place the muffins in the oven and bake for 30 minutes.

Let it cool for 10 minutes. Serve warm.

This recipe makes 12 servings.

Nutrition: 92 calories; 4g carbohydrates; 7g fats; 3g protein

Stir-Fried Vegetable Noodles

Dinner

Ingredients:

½ yellow onion, thinly sliced

2 large zucchinis

2 carrots

1 green bell pepper, thinly sliced

2 heads bok choy, sliced thinly

2 tablespoons olive oil

2 teaspoons garlic powder

1 teaspoon turmeric powder

4 tablespoons coconut aminos

2 tablespoons coconut sugar

Directions:

Use a spiralizer to slice zucchini and carrots into thin, long strands. Cut them further into 3-inch strands. Set aside.

Dissolve the sugar in coconut aminos. Set aside.

Heat the oil in a large pan over medium-high flame. Once the oil is hot, add in bell peppers, carrots, onions and half of the coconut aminos mixture. Cook for 5 minutes.

Add in zucchini, bok choy, garlic powder, turmeric powder and remaining coconut aminos. Stir-fry the ingredients for about 7 minutes. Serve warm.

This recipe makes 4 servings.

Nutrition: 160 calories; 20g carbohydrates; 7g fats; 7g protein

Caramel Coconut Truffles

Dessert

Ingredients:

Truffles:

2 ½ tablespoons coconut oil, melted

3 ½ tablespoons coconut sugar

3 ½ tablespoons cocoa powder

2 tablespoons coconut milk

2 ½ tablespoon butter, softened

Coating:

2 ½ tablespoons coconut sugar

1/8 teaspoon vanilla

2 ½ tablespoons butter

2 tablespoons coconut milk

1 cup desiccated coconut

Directions:

To make the truffles, combine coconut oil, coconut sugar, cocoa powder, coconut milk and butter, and mix well. Spoon the mixture into small round molds and freeze for 15 minutes.

While the truffles are setting, heat the butter in a saucepan over medium flame. Add coconut sugar and coconut milk then stir. Wait for the mixture to caramelize and bubble before adding the vanilla. Remove the caramel mixture from the heat and set aside.

Once the truffles are set, remove them from the molds. Pierce each truffle with a fork or skewer then dip it into the caramel. Roll the dipped truffles on the desiccated coconut and place it on a parchment-lined sheet.

Chill the truffles in the fridge for 1 hour then transfer them in an airtight container.

This recipe makes 10 servings

Nutrition: 100 calories; 1g carbohydrates; 11g fats; 0g protein

Day 2 - Eggs and Tomato Breakfast Skillet

Breakfast

Ingredients:

5 large eggs

½ cup chopped zucchini

½ chicken breast, boiled and chopped

2 garlic cloves, minced

½ cup chopped red bell pepper

1 small onion, minced

1 ½ cup pureed tomatoes

1 cup fresh basil leaves, torn

1 tablespoon olive oil

Pinch of salt and ground black pepper

Directions:

Heat the oil in a skillet over medium-high flame. Cook garlic and onions until onions are translucent. Add bell peppers and stir-fry for 5 minutes.

Stir in the chopped zucchini and chicken then cook for 6 minutes. Pour in tomato sauce then season with salt, pepper and basil leaves. Cook the dish for another 6 minutes with constant stirring.

Break each egg onto the sausage and veggie mixture, making sure to arrange the eggs neatly beside each other. Lower the flame to medium-low then cover the skillet.

Cook the dish for 10-12 minutes or until the eggs have set. Serve immediately.

This recipe makes 5 servings.

Nutrition: 220 calories; 5g carbohydrates; 16g fats; 9g protein

Mixed Greens and Mushrooms Soup

Lunch

Ingredients:

500 grams kale leaves, washed

250 grams spinach leaves, washed

250 grams collard greens, washed

1 cup button mushrooms, chopped

2 carrots, peeled and diced

1 yellow onion, chopped

1 tablespoon minced garlic

6 cups homemade chicken stock

2 teaspoons oregano powder

1 teaspoon thyme

3 tablespoons nutritional yeast

1 tablespoon butter

½ cup chopped basil

1 tablespoon lemon juice

Pinch of salt and ground black pepper

Directions:

Combine chicken stock, garlic, carrots and onions in a pot over medium-high heat. Simmer for 40 minutes.

Add in the kale, spinach, collard greens, mushrooms, lemon juice, nutritional yeast, basil and butter then stir. Season the soup mixture with oregano, thyme, salt and pepper. Simmer for 20-25 minutes or until the greens are completely cooked.

Turn off the heat and let the soup cool for 10 minutes. Use an immersion blender to cream the soup until you reach your desired consistency. Pour into bowls and serve while hot.

This recipe makes 4 servings.

Nutrition: 290 calories; 50g carbohydrates; 4g fats; 18g protein

Herbed Carrot Fritters

Snack

Ingredients:

700 grams carrots, peeled and sliced into fries

2 tablespoons olive oil

1 tablespoon dried rosemary

1 teaspoon cumin powder

2 garlic cloves, minced

Pinch of salt and ground black pepper

Directions:

Preheat the oven to 425° and grease a baking sheet with cooking spray.

Combine carrots, olive oil, rosemary, cumin, garlic, salt and pepper in a bowl and toss them together.

Place the carrots on the baking sheet and place in the oven. Bake for 10-15 minutes or until brown and tender. Let the fritters cool for 5 minutes then serve immediately.

This recipe makes 4 servings.

Nutrition: 130 calories; 17g carbohydrates; 7g fat; 2g protein

Almond-Crusted Crab Cakes with Balsamic Green Beans

Dinner

Ingredients:

450 grams fresh crabmeat

1 egg

1 teaspoon Dijon mustard

2 tablespoons mayonnaise

½ cup almond flour

¼ teaspoon lemon juice

¼ teaspoon chili powder

3 tablespoons coconut aminos

1 tablespoon finely chopped almonds

1 tablespoon chopped fresh parsley

2 teaspoons minced green onions

500 grams green beans, trimmed

Paleo Diet For Beginners

1 tablespoon balsamic vinegar

2 teaspoons minced garlic

2 tablespoons clarified butter

Directions:

Coat a baking sheet with cooking spray and preheat the oven to 400°F.

Combine chopped almonds and half of the almond flour in a bowl and set aside.

Whisk together egg, mustard, mayonnaise, lemon juice, 1 tablespoon coconut aminos, chili powder and remaining almond flour. Gradually add the crabmeat, parsley and green onions. Mix well or use your hands to knead the mixture.

Form 6 crabmeat patties from the mixture. Dredge each patty into the chopped almond breading.

Lay the patties on the baking sheet and place it in the oven. Bake for 20 minutes.

While the crab cakes are baking, heat the clarified butter in a pan over medium flame.

Sauté the garlic until it turns golden brown. Add in the green beans, balsamic vinegar, coconut aminos and water. Cover the pan and let it cook for 5 minutes.

Place the crab cakes on individual dinner plates and serve with a side of beans.

This recipe makes 6 servings.

Nutrition: 130 calories; 8g carbohydrates; 7g fats; 10g protein

Low-Carb Almond Chocolate Cookies

Dessert

Ingredients:

2 large eggs

1 ½ cups almond butter

¼ teaspoon salt

1 cup cocoa powder

¾ cup coconut sugar

Directions:

Preheat the oven to 325°F and prepare a parchment-lined cookie sheet.

Mix together the eggs, almond butter, salt, cocoa powder and powdered sugar in a bowl. Use a wooden spoon or a handheld mixer to blend the ingredients thoroughly.

Place 12 dough balls from the mixture and arrange them on the baking sheet. Gently press each ball with a fork to flatten it.

Place the cookie sheet in the oven and bake the dessert for 12-15 minutes. Let the cookies cool in a wire rack for 10 minutes before serving.

This recipe makes 12 serving.

Nutrition: 220 calories; 3g carbohydrates; 14g fats; 7g protein

Day 3 - Paleo Banana Pancake

Breakfast

Ingredients:

3 large eggs

¼ cup almond flour

1 banana, peeled and mashed

1/8 teaspoon baking soda

½ teaspoon cinnamon powder

1/8 teaspoon baking powder

1 teaspoon vanilla extract

1 tablespoon almond butter

2 teaspoons olive oil, melted

Directions:

Combine eggs, banana, flour, baking soda, baking powder, cinnamon, vanilla extract and almond butter in a bowl and whisk them together.

Heat the olive oil in a pan over medium-high flame. Pour a huge tablespoon of the batter into the pan and let the pancake cook for 3 minutes. Flip the pancake over and cook the other side for another 3 minutes.

Serve the pancakes with a side of honey.

This recipe makes 4 servings.

Nutrition: 120 calories; 8g carbohydrates; 7g fats; 6g protein

Tomato and Tuna Baskets

Lunch

Ingredients:

4 medium tomatoes

4 teaspoons nutritional yeast

1 tablespoon chopped celery

1 ½ cup canned tuna, drained and flaked

2 teaspoons lime juice

½ tablespoon mustard

2 ½ tablespoons mayonnaise

½ teaspoon chopped parsley

Pinch of sea salt and ground black pepper

Directions:

Slice 1/3 of the tomatoes off and use the bottom part. Scoop out the seeds and pulp and let the tomatoes drain. Set aside.

Preheat the oven to 375°F and prepare a small

baking dish.

Combine tuna, celery, mayonnaise, lime juice, mustard, salt and pepper in a bowl and mix well. Scoop the tuna mixture into each tomato basket.

Sprinkle equal portions of nutritional yeast and parsley on top of each tomato basket then arrange them inside the baking dish. Bake for 15 minutes and serve.

This recipe makes 4 servings.

Nutrition: 170 calories; 4g carbohydrates; 12g fats; 13g protein

Roasted Broccoli Bites

Snack

Ingredients:

1 kilogram broccoli florets, halved

½ teaspoon ground black pepper

3 garlic cloves, crushed

2 ½ teaspoons olive oil

1 teaspoon sea salt

Directions:

Preheat the oven to 400°F and line a baking sheet with parchment paper.

Place the broccoli florets, olive oil and garlic in a bowl. Season it with salt and pepper then toss.

Arrange the vegetables on the baking sheet. Bake the broccoli in the oven for 30 minutes. Let it cool for 5-10 minutes then serve immediately.

This recipe makes 6 servings.

Nutrition: 75 calories; 12g carbohydrates; 3g fats; 5g protein

Fiery Curried Chicken with Sautéed Broccoli

Dinner

Ingredients:
600 grams chicken breast, deboned
1 ½ cups coconut milk
2 teaspoons minced ginger
¾ teaspoon turmeric
¾ teaspoon curry powder
1 teaspoon minced garlic
¾ teaspoon cumin
1 jalapeno, chopped
½ teaspoon cinnamon powder
1 teaspoon salt
½ teaspoon ground black pepper
Juice from 1 lime
4 basil leaves, chopped
2 cups broccoli florets
1 tablespoon olive oil
1 teaspoon garlic powder
1 teaspoon sesame seeds

Directions:

Place basil, lime juice, pepper, salt, cinnamon powder, jalapeno, cumin, turmeric, curry

powder, garlic, ginger and coconut milk in a blender. Process the curry sauce until the spices have blended into the milk.
Arrange the chicken pieces inside the slow cooker. Pour the blended curry sauce on the chicken and cover the pot.
Cook the chicken on high for 4 hours.

Note: If you don't have a slow cooker, you can also use the stovetop method to prepare this recipe. Just add two tablespoons of olive oil in a saucepan and brown the chicken pieces.

Pour in the prepared curry sauce together with half a cup of water then cover it. Let the dish simmer over medium flame for 30-40 minutes or until the chicken pieces are tender. Stir the dish every 5 minutes while cooking it.

While the chicken is cooking, heat the olive oil in a pan over medium-high flame. Add in broccoli and garlic powder then sauté for 5 minutes. Once the vegetables are tender, turn off the flame then sprinkle sesame seeds on top of the broccoli.

Place the cooked curry in individual bowls then serve it with a side of broccoli.
This recipe makes 4 servings.

Nutrition: 250 calories; 7g carbohydrates; 6g fats; 35g protein

Chewy Lemon Tartlets

Dessert

Ingredients:

9 tablespoons fresh lemon juice

1 cup almond flour

3 dates, pitted and chopped

2 eggs, whisked

1 teaspoon lemon zest

1 tablespoon coconut sugar

1 teaspoon water

Directions:

Preheat the oven to 350°F and prepare 4 muffin tins with cupcake liners.

For the crust, place 3 tablespoons of the lemon juice, almond flour and dates in a food processor. Grind the ingredients together then spoon equal amounts inside the muffin tins. Press the mixture down and sideways. Bake the crust in the oven for 12 minutes.

While the crust is baking, prepare the lemon filling. Pour the remaining lemon juice, coconut sugar, water and zest in a saucepan over low flame. Stir the mixture over the heat for 2 minutes.

Slowly pour in the eggs while the lemon mixture is simmering. Whisk vigorously then turn off the heat. Let the lemon mixture cool at room temperature for 5 minutes.

Pour the lemon mixture into the baked crust. Chill the tartlets inside the fridge for 1 hour. Serve immediately.

This recipe makes 4 servings.

Nutrition: 240 calories; 20g carbohydrates; 16g fats; 9g protein

Day 4 - Savoury Turkey and Veggie Frittata

Breakfast

Ingredients:

6 eggs

1 cup chopped turkey meat, pre-cooked

2 medium tomatoes, deseeded and sliced

2 tablespoons green chopped onions

½ cup chopped zucchini

½ cup sliced olives

8 basil leaves

½ red bell pepper, chopped

Pinch of salt and ground black pepper

Directions:

Preheat the oven to 350°F and lightly grease a 9-inch round baking dish.

Whisk together eggs, salt and pepper. Set aside.

Layer the ingredients inside the baking dish in this order: turkey meat, tomatoes, green onions, basil, zucchini, olives and bell pepper. Gradually pour the whisked eggs into the dish.

Place the dish in the oven and bake the frittata for 30 minutes. Once done, let it cool for 10 minutes. Slice and serve.

This recipe makes 6 servings.

Nutrition: 190 calories; 4g carbohydrates; 18g fat; 10g protein

Spicy Barbecued Shrimp Skewers

Lunch

Ingredients:

550 grams shrimp, peeled and deveined

¼ teaspoon cayenne pepper

2 teaspoons paprika

¼ teaspoon dried oregano

¼ teaspoon dried thyme

1 teaspoon garlic powder

½ teaspoon ground black pepper

½ teaspoon salt

1 tablespoon olive oil

1 teaspoon onion powder

Wood skewers (pre-soaked in water)

Directions:

Preheat the barbecue grill to medium-high temperature.

Combine the shrimps with the olive oil, salt, pepper, onion powder, garlic powder, thyme, cayenne pepper, oregano and paprika. Toss the ingredients until all the shrimps are evenly coated.

Get a wooden skewer and thread 3-4 shrimps. Do the same procedure for all the shrimps.

Place the shrimps on the grill and roast for 3 minutes per side. Serve immediately.

This recipe makes 4 servings.

Nutrition: 180 calories; 2g carbohydrates; 1g fats; 30g protein

15-Minute Granola Bars

Snack

Ingredients:
½ cup coconut flakes
2 tablespoons sunflower seeds
½ cup almonds
2 tablespoon sesame seeds
2 tablespoons almond butter
3 ½ tablespoons coconut sugar
1 large egg
1 teaspoon cinnamon powder
1 tablespoon molasses
1 teaspoon vanilla extract
Pinch of sea salt

Directions:

Preheat the oven to 350°F and lightly grease a
9 x 5 loaf pan.

Place coconut flakes, sunflower seeds,
almonds, sesame seeds, almond butter,
coconut sugar, egg, cinnamon powder,
molasses, vanilla and salt in a food processor.
Mix until the ingredients are finely ground.

Transfer the mixture into the loaf pan. Press the granola mixture downwards into the pan to make it more compact.

Bake the granola for 15 minutes. Slice into 6 equal portions then let it cool at room temperature. You can serve it immediately or place it in the fridge. This recipe makes 6 servings.

Nutrition: 170 calories; 10g carbohydrates; 12g fats; 5g protein

Chicken Adobo in a Crockpot with Mango Salsa

Dinner

Ingredients:

4 skinless chicken thighs

2 skinless chicken breasts, halved

5 garlic cloves, crushed

1 large onion, chopped

2 bay leaves

½ cup coconut aminos

¾ cup apple cider vinegar

2 teaspoons paprika

½ teaspoon black peppercorns

1 tablespoon coconut sugar

2 unripe mangoes, diced

4 tomatoes, chopped

½ cup chopped cilantro

1 red onion, sliced

1 tablespoon lemon juice

Directions:

Place the chicken thighs, breast halves, garlic and onions inside the crockpot. Pour in coconut aminos and apple cider vinegar. Season the chicken with coconut sugar, peppercorns, bay leaves and paprika.

Cover the crock pot then cook the dish on high temperature for 4 hours.

Note: If you don't have a crock pot, try the stovetop method. Just sauté the garlic and onions in a pot with some olive oil. Once the onions become translucent, add in the chicken pieces, coconut aminos, vinegar, peppercorns, bay leaf and paprika. Cover the pot and let it simmer over medium-high flame for 45-50 minutes.

While the adobo is cooking, place the mangoes, tomatoes, cilantro, onions and lemon juice in a bowl and toss them together.

Chill the salsa in the fridge until the adobo is ready to serve.

Once the adobo is cooked, transfer the chicken pieces into a serving bowl then pour the adobo sauce over it. Serve the mango salsa together with the adobo dish.

This recipe makes 4 servings.

Nutrition: 450 calories; 20g carbohydrates; 22g fats; 40g protein

Spicy Chocolate Squares

Dessert

Ingredients:

½ cup cocoa powder

½ teaspoon almond extract

½ cup coconut oil

3 tablespoons honey

1 teaspoon cayenne pepper

1 tablespoon chopped almonds

Directions:

Heat the coconut oil in a saucepan over medium-high flame. Once the coconut oil is heated, mix in cocoa powder, almond extract, honey and cayenne pepper. Mix well.

Turn off the heat then fold in the chopped almonds into the melted chocolate. Pour the chocolate into molds and freeze for 1 hour.

This recipe makes 6 servings.

Nutrition: 160 calories; 11g carbohydrates; 15g fats; 2g protein

Day 5 - Green and Red Scrambled Eggs

Breakfast

Ingredients:

8 large eggs, whisked

2 cups frozen spinach, thawed and chopped

1 red bell pepper, deseeded and chopped

1 large tomato, diced

½ cup white onion, minced

1 avocado, pitted, peeled and sliced

Pinch of sea salt and ground black pepper

1 tablespoon olive oil

Directions:

Heat the olive oil in a pan over medium-high heat.

Place the spinach, bell pepper, onion and tomato in the pan and cook for 4 minutes.

Once the vegetables are tender, pour in the eggs and cook it for 4-5 minutes.

Whisk the eggs constantly while cooking to make it fluffy. Season the eggs with salt and pepper.

Transfer the scrambled eggs on a plate and serve it with avocado slices on top.

This recipe makes 5 servings.

Nutrition: 280 calories; 12g carbohydrates; 20g fats; 15g protein

Buttered Vegetable Rice

Lunch

Ingredients:

8 medium carrots, peeled and chopped

1 large cauliflower head, chopped

¼ cup water

3 tablespoons butter

2 teaspoons turmeric

Pinch of sea salt and black ground pepper

Directions:

Place the carrots and cauliflower in a food processor and pulse until the vegetables are finely chopped.

Transfer the chopped vegetables from the food processor to a skillet. Pour water into the skillet and cook on medium-low heat for 25 minutes. Stir the vegetables then drain the water completely. Turn off the flame.

On a smaller pan, melt the butter until golden brown. Mix in the turmeric then pour the butter mixture onto the vegetable rice. Season with salt and pepper then toss the ingredients together. Serve immediately.

This recipe makes 8-10 servings.

Nutrition: 90 calories; 12g carbohydrates; 4g fats; 3g protein

Banana Raspberry Cooler

Snack

Ingredients:

2 cups raspberries

3 bananas, peeled and chopped

1 tablespoon coconut oil

1 tablespoons flaxseed meal

2 tablespoons finely ground almonds

2 cups water

2 cups coconut milk

2 teaspoons coconut sugar

Directions:

Combine raspberries, bananas, coconut oil, coconut milk, water, coconut sugar, almonds and flaxseed in a blender. Process for 1 minute then pour in individual glasses.

This recipe makes 4 servings.

Nutrition: 304 calories; 55g carbohydrates; 14g fats; 4g protein

Beef and Vegetable Stew with Mashed Parsnip

Dinner

Ingredients:

680 grams beef stew meat, cubed

1 ½ cups cauliflower florets

1 ½ cups chopped zucchini

1 white onion, quartered

2 tablespoons butter

1 ½ cup pureed tomatoes

1 ½ cup water

1 tablespoon coconut aminos

½ teaspoon lemon pepper seasoning

3 parsnips, peeled and boiled

¾ cup almond milk

2 tablespoons olive oil

Pinch of sea salt

Directions:

Arrange the beef cubes at the bottom of the crockpot. Add in cauliflower, zucchini, onions and butter.

Combine coconut aminos, pureed tomatoes and water in a bowl and mix well. Pour the tomato mixture into the crockpot. Season the dish with lemon pepper seasoning.

Cover the pot and set the temperature to low. Let the beef stew cook for 8 hours.

Note: You can also use the stovetop method for this recipe. Just heat the butter in a pot over medium-high flame then brown the beef cubes. Add in coconut aminos, onions, tomatoes and water. Cover the pot then simmer for 2 hours. Once the beef is tender, add in cauliflower and zucchini then cook for another 30 minutes.

While the beef stew is cooking, dice the boiled parsnips then place them in a bowl. Start mashing the parsnips with a fork or a potato masher while slowly pouring in the olive oil and almond milk. Continue mashing the vegetable until the texture becomes smooth and creamy. Season the dish with sea salt.

Transfer the beef stew to a large bowl then place the mashed parsnip on a serving plate. Serve immediately.

This recipe makes 6 servings.

Nutrition: 280 calories; 20g carbohydrates; 15g fats; 25g protein

Creamy Coconut Pudding

Dessert

Ingredients:

2 ½ cups coconut milk

¼ cup cocoa powder

1 tablespoon shredded coconut

¼ cup honey

1 teaspoon coconut sugar

1 teaspoon vanilla extract

Pinch of salt

1 cup chia seeds

Directions:

Place 2 cups coconut milk, honey, cocoa powder, salt and vanilla in a bowl and whisk them together. Mix in chia seeds. Cover the bowl with plastic wrap then chill in the fridge for 8 hours. This will allow the pudding to thicken.

In a small bowl, mix together the coconut sugar and shredded coconut. Set aside.

Spoon the chilled coconut pudding into individual bowls. Pour the remaining coconut milk into each bowl then sprinkle the sugar and shredded coconut mixture on top. Serve immediately.

This recipe makes 6 servings.

Nutrition: 205 calories; 15g carbohydrates; 16g fats; 3g

Day 6 - Chicken Breakfast Patties

Breakfast

Ingredients:

500 grams ground chicken

½ teaspoon ground black pepper

2 teaspoons salt

½ teaspoon paprika

1 teaspoon dried sage

1 teaspoon turmeric powder

¼ teaspoon dried marjoram

½ teaspoon dried oregano

½ teaspoon coconut sugar

3 tablespoons olive oil

Directions:

Place the ground chicken in a bowl. Season the

meat with salt, pepper, oregano, sage, marjoram, turmeric, paprika and sugar. Mix well then place in the fridge for 3-4 hours.

Take out the chilled sausage mixture. Create 8 balls from the mixture and flatten them to create patties. Set aside.

Heat the oil in a pan over medium-high flame. Lay the patties on the pan and cook each side for 5 minutes. Place the breakfast patties on a serving plate and serve immediately.

This recipe makes 8 servings.

Nutrition: 150 calories; 1g carbohydrates; 12g fats; 10g protein

Fried Okra and Chicken Salad

Lunch

Ingredients:

450 grams frozen okra, sliced

1 small chicken breast, boiled and chopped

½ cup chopped red bell pepper

1 small onion, chopped

1 small tomato, diced

2 tablespoons coconut sugar

2 tablespoons balsamic vinegar

2 tablespoons olive oil

Directions:

Whisk together coconut sugar, olive oil and balsamic vinegar. Chill the dressing in the fridge.

Place the chopped chicken breast in a pan over medium-high flame and cook until brown.

Remove the chicken from the pan and set aside.

Add the okra pieces into the pan and cook for 5 minutes. Turn off the heat then add the onion, tomatoes and bell peppers. Mix well.

Transfer the okra salad into a bowl then pour in the balsamic dressing. Add in the chicken then toss the salad. Chill the salad for 1 hour then serve.

This recipe makes 4 servings.

Nutrition: 220 calories; 20g carbohydrates; 16g fats; 3g protein

Gluten Free Almond Cookies

Snack

Ingredients:

½ cup almond flour

1/3 cup coconut sugar

¼ cup slivered almonds

1 egg white

½ teaspoon almond extract

Directions:

Preheat the oven to 300°F and prepare a parchment-lined baking dish.

Whisk together egg white, coconut sugar and almond extract. Fold in almond flour and slivered almonds. Mix well.

Pour the cookie mixture into the 8 x 8 baking dish and spread evenly. Place it in the oven and bake for 25 minutes.

Let the baked cookie mixture cool at room

temperature for 10 minutes. Use a knife to slice the cookie mixture into squares. Serve warm.

This recipe makes 8 servings.

Nutrition: 30 calories; 5g carbohydrates; 1g fats; 1g protein

Spice-Rubbed Salmon Fillet with Herbed Tomato Salad

Dinner

Ingredients:

4 medium salmon fillets

2 tablespoons olive oil

½ teaspoon dried oregano

½ teaspoon ground black pepper

½ teaspoon sea salt

1 tablespoon paprika

¼ teaspoon chili powder

½ teaspoon onion powder

2 cups cherry tomatoes, halved

2 tablespoons chopped mint

2 tablespoons chopped parsley

1 tablespoon lemon juice

2 teaspoons balsamic vinegar

Directions:

Combine oregano, pepper, salt, paprika, chili powder and onion powder in a bowl. Place the salmon fillets into the bowl of spices and toss until the fillets are evenly coated.

Heat a tablespoon of oil in a grill pan over medium-high flame. Place the salmon fillets skin down on the pan and cook for 4 minutes. Flip the fish over and cook the other side for another 4 minutes.

Place the fillets on a plate and let it cool.

To make the salad, whisk together the remaining oil, lemon juice and balsamic vinegar. Add in the tomatoes, parsley and mint then toss the salad.

Arrange each fillet on a dinner plate together with a side of tomato salad. Serve immediately.

This recipe makes 4 servings.

Nutrition: 300 calories; 5g carbohydrates; 14g fats; 35g protein

Lime and Watermelon Sorbet
Dessert

Ingredients:

4 cups deseeded watermelon cubes

¾ cup fresh lime juice

3 cups coconut sugar

3 cups water

Directions:

Puree the watermelon cubes in a food processor. Set aside.

Combine water and coconut sugar in a saucepan over medium flame. Stir until the sugar dissolves and the mixture starts to simmer. Turn off the flame then pour the syrup mixture into a bowl.

Mix in the lime juice and pureed watermelon into the bowl of syrup. Stir the sorbet mixture then let it cool for 1 hour in the fridge.

Pour the sorbet mixture into an ice cream

maker and process until it reaches a soft consistency. Transfer the sorbet into an airtight container and place in the freezer overnight.

This recipe makes 10 servings.

Nutrition: 300 calories; 70g carbohydrates; 0g fats; 1g protein

Day 7 - Grain-Free Morning Cereal

Breakfast

Ingredients:

2 apples, cored and diced

2 bananas

3 eggs

½ cup ground pecans

2 tablespoons coconut sugar

½ cup coconut milk

1 teaspoon cinnamon powder

1 teaspoon coconut oil

2 tablespoons almond butter

1 tablespoon flaxseed meal

Directions:

Place diced apples, cinnamon powder and

coconut oil in a saucepan over medium flame. Cook for 5 minutes.

While the apples are cooking, process banana, pecans, eggs, flaxseed, coconut milk and almond butter in a food processor. Blend until the ingredients are finely ground and creamy.

Pour the banana nut mixture into the apples and stir. Simmer the cereal for 10 minutes then remove from heat. Serve in individual bowls.

This recipe makes 4 servings.

Nutrition: 360 calories; 20g carbohydrates; 30g fats; 13g protein

Spicy Steak and Lettuce Tacos Lunch

Ingredients:

250 grams flank steak

6 Romaine lettuce leaves

½ teaspoon ground black pepper

½ teaspoon sea salt

½ teaspoon cumin

¼ teaspoon paprika

1 tablespoon lemon juice

12 avocado slices

6 tablespoons chopped tomatoes

6 teaspoons chopped cilantro

Directions:

Place the flank steak in a bowl then sprinkle it with sea salt, pepper, cumin, paprika and lemon juice. Rub the spices all over the meat and let it marinade in the fridge for 2 hours.

Preheat the grilling pan over medium-high flame. Place the marinated steak on the grill pan and cook each side for 5 minutes. Let the steak rest for 10 minutes on the chopping board.

Slice the steak into strips and place them on top of the lettuce leaves. Place 2 avocado slices, a tablespoon of tomatoes and a teaspoon of cilantro on top of each portion of lettuce and steak. Serve immediately.

This recipe makes 6 servings.

Nutrition: 170 calories; 1g carbohydrates; 6g fats; 24g protein

Almond Sesame Crackers

Snack

Ingredients:

¾ cup ground almonds

¾ cup almond flour

1 large egg white

½ tablespoon sesame seeds

½ tablespoon olive oil

½ teaspoon sea salt

2 tablespoons water

¼ teaspoon garlic powder

Directions:

Preheat the oven to 350°F and lightly grease a flat baking sheet with cooking spray.

Combine ground almond, almond flour, egg white, sesame seeds, water, and garlic powder in a bowl. Knead with your hands until a soft dough forms.

Place the dough in between 2 wax papers and lay it on the baking sheet. Use a rolling pin to flatten out the dough slowly until it becomes a quarter of an inch thick. Chill the flattened dough in the fridge for 10 minutes.

Gently peel the wax paper on both sides of the dough then use a knife to score the dough into 10 equal portions.

Brush olive oil on the surface of the dough then sprinkle sea salt on top. Bake the dough for 15 minutes or until the surface turns brown. Remove from oven and let it cool for 10 minutes.

This recipe makes 10 servings.

Nutrition: 250 calories; 5g carbohydrates; 10g fats; 10g protein

Sweet and Spicy Gingered Chicken with Roasted Brussels Sprouts

Dinner

Ingredients:

680 grams chicken breasts, halved

500 grams Brussels sprouts

½ teaspoon red pepper flakes

1 tablespoon honey

2 tablespoons coconut aminos

½ cup pureed tomatoes

½ cup homemade chicken stock

½ cup pureed peaches

1 tablespoon sesame oil

1 tablespoon grated fresh ginger

¼ cup minced onion

2 garlic cloves, minced

1 small red bell pepper, deseeded and chopped

1 tablespoon olive oil

2 tablespoons lemon juice

¼ cup toasted sesame seeds, chopped

Directions:

Combine pepper flakes, honey, coconut aminos, tomato puree, apricot puree, sesame oil, ginger, onion and garlic in a 6-quart crockpot and stir. Pour in the chicken broth and mix well.

Place the chicken pieces into the pot then sprinkle chopped bell peppers on top. Cover the pot and set the crockpot on high. Cook for 4 hours.

While the chicken is cooking, slice the Brussels sprouts in half then place them on a baking dish. Pour the olive oil and lemon juice over the vegetables then place them in the oven. Bake the vegetables for 30 minutes under 300°F.

Remove the chicken from the pot and transfer to a bowl. Pour the sauce over the dish then arrange the roasted Brussels sprouts around it. Serve immediately.

This recipe makes 5 servings.

Nutrition: 260 calories; 25g carbohydrates; 20g fats; 29g protein

Moist Pineapple Upside-Down Cake Dessert

Ingredients:

5 slices fresh pineapple rings

½ cup pineapple juice

½ cup almond flour

½ cup coconut flour

2 tablespoons butter

2 ½ tablespoons coconut sugar

1 ½ tablespoons shredded coconut

½ cup organic honey

1 teaspoon almond extract

2 large eggs

1 medium banana, mashed

1 ½ teaspoon baking powder

Directions:

Preheat the oven to 375°F and coat a 9-inch round cake pan with cooking spray.

Place the butter into the cake pan and melt it in the oven for 2 minutes. Once the butter melts, take the pan out of the oven. Sprinkle coconut sugar and shredded coconut into the bottom of the pan then neatly arrange the pineapple slices. Set aside.

Combine almond flour, coconut flour and baking powder in a bowl and mix well. Set aside.

In a separate bowl, mix together eggs, banana, honey, pineapple juice and almond extract. Add this wet mixture into the flour mixture. Mix thoroughly.

Pour the batter into the cake pan, covering the pineapple rings. Bake it in the oven for 45 minutes.

Remove the pan from the oven and loosen the sides of the cake with a knife. Place a large plate on top of the cake pan and slowly flip the cake over. Slice before serving.

This recipe makes 6 servings.

Nutrition: 240 calories, 32g carbohydrates; 11g fats; 6g protein

Try out this 7-day Paleo meal challenge: you will be amazed at how delicious organic food can be and, after a few days, you will see positive changes manifesting in your body, mind and spirit. Moreover, the wide selection of Paleo-friendly ingredients encourages creativity and enjoyment while cooking in the kitchen.

Enjoy the recipes!

Extra Paleo Recipes for your Meal Plan – Low-Calorie Sautéed Mushrooms

To add variety to your week-long healthy meal plan, here are 7 more recipes that you can incorporate into your new Paleo lifestyle. These recipes contain the most colorful, organic and nutritious ingredients that will help you achieve alertness, agility and a fitter body.

Low-Calorie Sautéed Mushrooms

Ingredients:

800 grams button mushrooms, halved

1½ tablespoons balsamic vinegar

1 tablespoon ghee

1 tablespoon minced garlic

1 teaspoon chopped fresh parsley

1 tablespoon olive oil

Pinch of sea salt and ground black pepper

Directions:

Heat the ghee and olive oil in a pan over medium-high flame. Cook the mushrooms in the pan for 3 minutes or until tender.

Lower the flame to medium. Add in garlic, vinegar, salt and pepper. Stir while cooking for 2 minutes. Turn off the heat then transfer the mushrooms to a plate.

Sprinkle chopped parsley on top then serve.

This recipe makes 6 servings.

Nutrition: 85 calories; 5g carbohydrates; 7g fats; 4g protein

Roasted Summer Salad

Ingredients:

1 cup cherry tomatoes, halved

1 large zucchini, sliced

1 white onion, chopped

2 summer squash, chopped

1 yellow bell pepper, deseeded and chopped

1 eggplant, sliced

2 tablespoons lemon juice

3 tablespoons olive oil

1 teaspoon honey

Pinch of sea salt and ground black pepper

Directions:

To make the dressing, whisk the lemon juice, olive oil, honey, salt and pepper together until smooth. Set aside.

Grease a large grill pan with the remaining

olive oil. Lay the tomatoes, zucchini, onion, summer squash, bell pepper and eggplant slices on the pan and roast them over high flame for 5-7 minutes. Once the vegetables have grill marks underneath, flip them over and grill for another 7 minutes.

Turn off the heat then let the vegetables cool at room temperature for 5 minutes.

Transfer the roasted vegetables in a bowl then pour in the dressing. Toss the salad then chill it in the fridge for 1 hour.

This recipe makes 4 servings.

Nutrition: 140 calories; 17g carbohydrates; 8g fats; 4g protein

Paleo Pumpkin Loaf

Ingredients:

4 large eggs

5 tablespoons coconut oil, melted

2 cups almond flour

1 ½ cup pureed pumpkin

4 teaspoons pumpkin spice

1 teaspoon sea salt

1 ½ teaspoons baking powder

1 ½ teaspoons baking soda

½ cup honey

2 teaspoons vanilla extract

Directions:

Preheat the oven to 350°F and prepare a 9 x 5 loaf pan lined with parchment paper.

Combine almond flour, sea salt, pumpkin spice, baking soda and baking powder in a bowl. Set aside.

In a separate bowl, whisk the eggs, honey, coconut oil and vanilla extract together. Slowly pour in the pureed pumpkin and mix well.

Fold the wet ingredients into the dry ingredients and blend until the bread batter becomes moist. Pour the mixture into the prepared loaf pan.

Bake the loaf in the oven for 20 minutes. Let the bread cool for 10 minutes before slicing into it.

This recipe makes 8 servings.

Nutrition: 250 calories; 25g carbohydrates; 13g fats; 6g protein

Creamy Avocado and Butternut Soup

Ingredients:

2 cups sliced butternut squash, peeled

1 small red onion, minced

1 cup mashed avocado meat

3 cups homemade chicken stock

1 tablespoon coconut oil

3 tablespoons almond milk

1 tablespoon cinnamon powder

1 tablespoon nutmeg

1 tablespoon cayenne pepper

2 teaspoons turmeric powder

2 teaspoons honey

Directions:

Heat the oil in a pot over medium-high flame. Add the chopped onions and cook for 7 minutes.

Add in the honey, turmeric powder, cayenne pepper, nutmeg and cinnamon powder then stir. Gradually add the butternut squash and mashed avocado then cook for 5 minutes.

Pour in the almond milk and chicken stock. Cover the pot and simmer for 30 minutes or until the squash is tender.

Remove the soup from the heat. Use an immersion blender inside the pot and mix the ingredients together. Pour into individual bowls and serve immediately.

This recipe makes 8 servings.

Nutrition: 190 calories; 27g carbohydrates; 9g fats; 3g protein

Tossed Broccoli and Beef Salad

Ingredients:

150 grams cooked roast beef

1 ½ head broccoli, chopped into small florets

1 tablespoon lemon juice

1 small red onion, chopped

½ cup chopped almonds

1 cup mayonnaise

2 tablespoons honey

Pinch of black ground pepper

Directions:

To create the dressing, whisk together the lemon juice, mayonnaise, honey and ground black pepper. Set aside.

Shred the roast beef and place it in a bowl. Add in the broccoli, almonds and onions then mix. Pour in the prepared dressing then toss the salad. Place in fridge for 1 hour before serving.

This recipe makes 6 servings.

Nutrition: 250 calories; 18g carbohydrates; 25g fats; 7g protein

Paleo Spicy Beef Jerky

Ingredients:

1 ½ kilograms roast beef, thinly sliced into strips

1 cup coconut aminos

1 tablespoon onion powder

1 tablespoon paprika

½ cup hot water

1 ½ tablespoons garlic powder

2 teaspoons cayenne pepper

1 teaspoon chili powder

1 tablespoon coconut sugar

Directions:

Preheat the oven to 200°F and prepare a wire rack and a dripping pan at the bottom.

Whisk together coconut aminos, coconut sugar and hot water. Add in onion powder, garlic powder, paprika, cayenne pepper and chili powder. Stir the spices together.

Place the meat strips into the spice mixture and marinade for 8 hours. After 8 hours, drain the marinated meat completely. Hang the strips of meat on the wire rack, making sure to place the pan at the bottom in case oil and sauces drip.

Bake the beef strips for 5 hours. Let it cool at room temperature then transfer these to an airtight container.

This recipe makes 6 servings.

Nutrition: 70 calories; 8g carbohydrates; 3g fats; 3g protein

Almond Walnut Brownies

Ingredients:

½ cup chopped walnuts

½ cup almond flour, blanched

2 small eggs, whisked

1 ½ teaspoons vanilla extract

3 tablespoons coconut oil, melted

½ cup raw honey

3 tablespoons cocoa powder

Directions:

Preheat the oven to 325°F and prepare a 9 x 9 brownie pan by greasing it with cooking spray and dusting it with some almond flour.

Combine almond flour and cocoa powder in a bowl and mix well. Gradually add in the eggs, vanilla, coconut oil and honey. Blend the ingredients well. Fold in the chopped walnuts.

Pour the brownie batter into the pan and use a

spatula to spread the mixture to the sides. Bake the brownies in the oven for 25 minutes.

Once the brownies are done, let them cool for 10 minutes before slicing.

This recipe makes 6 servings.

Nutrition: 290 calories; 25g carbohydrates; 20g fats; 6g protein

Conclusion

Thank you again for purchasing this book!

I hope this book was able to motivate you to adopt a healthier lifestyle known as the Paleo Diet. After reading the chapters, it is expected that you now have full awareness and understanding of the connection between clean, organic food and one's physical, mental and emotional state.

In addition to that, the recipes in this book show how quick and easy it is to prepare organic dishes daily by using only the freshest, most nutritious and economical ingredients in the market. All it takes is commitment, careful planning and being mindful of healthier options when it comes to creating a paleo meal plan, which is free of sugars, grains and starches.

The delicious paleo recipes in this book were created for you to enjoy the processes of meal planning and cooking while transitioning into a healthier lifestyle. Once you start following the food guide, recipes and meal plans, you will eventually get used to the paleo way of living and sooner or later, you will find yourself reaping numerous health benefits that will improve the quality of your life.

The next step is to commit to a better lifestyle by continuing to cook the paleo recipes found in this book. You may even try creating your own version of these dishes by making small ingredient changes without straying from the diet's principles.

Finally, it is highly beneficial to use this book as a guide to making a positive and long-term change for your health. The principles and rules of the paleo diet will help you make smarter choices while shopping for ingredients. It can also further develop your appreciation for better nutrition and wellness. It is time to embrace a cleaner and organic lifestyle permanently by using all the information that you've learned from this book.

Finally, if you enjoyed this book, then I'd like to ask you for a favor, would you be kind

Paleo Diet For Beginners

Thank you and all the best!

If you enjoyed this book, why not check out my other books...

Preview Of 'Leptin Resistance Overcome: 17 Simple Steps To Fix Your Leptin Resistance, Beat Obesity, Get In Control of Your Weight and increase your Energy

Learn how to finally master your LEPTIN RESISTANCE, which will help you BURN FAT and BUILD MUSCLE all at the same time using the powerful and effective proven methods in this book today!

This book will help you see that your leptin resistance condition is not permanent. It CAN be overcome! Through careful action and persistent steps taken in the right direction, you CAN overcome your resistance to leptin. I am here to give you hope that you can still realize your dream of losing weight!

Let me ask you – are you tired of being overweight? Can you no longer stand obesity and all of the negative consequences that it brings? Have you already tried countless diets, exercise programs, and weight-loss programs in order to overcome it, but to little avail? And to crown it all, it has just been revealed to you that you are resistant to leptin – a hormone that causes a decrease in hunger at the end of a meal and helps to balance energy in the body. Enter this book...

This book will teach you all that you need know on the subject and how to start combating it. Through the years, much information has been gathered and a wealth of research and information that has investigated numerous methods of getting it under control. Doctors and health authorities have been consulted and have tried and tested many of the solutions they prescribed. And so, in this book, you will be presented with that great wealth of well researched information and solutions.

This book discusses in detail several solutions and cures that have worked for many. You will be pleased to hear that most of the cures described are simple changes that you can apply to your daily routine – all of them natural, safe, and healthy! Leptin resistance can definitely be overcome through natural methods (I know, because it worked for me and countless others!) and this is the core message that this book aims to deliver.

So take action and embark upon this journey of discovery and revelation. There is so much this book wants to share with you. There are so many wonderful suggestions and practical tips that you can start applying immediately. And if you do so, you will start seeing a beautiful change in your condition!

Start reading now, and start applying the techniques

today. You have nothing to lose but a whole lot of weight!

Here is a preview of what you will learn in this life changing book...

- What Leptin Actually Is
- How It Functions In Your Day
- What Leptin Resistance Is
- How To Beat The Resistance
- Do You Need To Supplement Leptin
- Symptoms Of Leptin Resistance
- Possible Causes Of Leptin Resistance
- And Much, much more!

Have a look at what others are saying about this book:

Brilliant book! It was very easy to read and helped me understand the importance of overcoming leptin resistance. I found this book particularly helpful because it was packed full of practical tips that I can apply straight away. It gave me a clear plan of what to do and I can't wait to start! It increased my motivation and confidence that I can definitely lead a healthy lifestyle. I loved how the book understood health challenges, and gave hope and help for a brighter future. Uzma

Grab your copy now and start your journey to a better you!

Check Out My Other Books

http://justreadme.com/

Bonus:

As promised here is the info to search your free gift's. I really hope you enjoy and they benefit you greatly. Thanks again!

http://justreadme.com/paleo-bonus/

Made in the USA
San Bernardino, CA
18 April 2018